T0193871

THE TRUTH ABOUT
BLOOD PRESSURE

THE TRUTH ABOUT BLOOD PRESSURE

THE MISINTERPRETATION

FRED A. WERKMEISTER E.E.

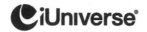

THE TRUTH ABOUT BLOOD PRESSURE
THE MISINTERPRETATION

iUniverse books may be ordered through booksellers or by contacting:

iUniverse
1663 Liberty Drive
Bloomington, IN 47403
www.iuniverse.com
1-800-Authors (1-800-288-4677)

Because of the dynamic nature of the Internet, any web addresses or links contained in this book may have changed since publication and may no longer be valid. The views expressed in this work are solely those of the author and do not necessarily reflect the views of the publisher, and the publisher hereby disclaims any responsibility for them.

Any people depicted in stock imagery provided by Getty Images are models, and such images are being used for illustrative purposes only. Certain stock imagery © Getty Images.

ISBN: 978-1-5320-6918-5 (sc)
ISBN: 978-1-5320-6919-2 (e)

Library of Congress Control Number: 2020904756

Print information available on the last page.

iUniverse rev. date: 03/27/2020

The heart has its reasons which reason knows nothing of...We know the truth not only by the reason, but by the heart.

- Blaise Pascal

CONTENTS

AUTHOR PREFACE

This book contains material collected from five years of research undertaken for personal reasons. I am an electrical engineer, author and researcher with extensive experience in industrial control systems. My cardiologist diagnosed me with hypertension and suggested that I read available literature to get a better understanding of what high blood pressure is. After reading hundreds of opinions in many books, I concluded that, like everyone else, I had a minimal and incorrect knowledge of what high blood pressure is, what causes it and why blood pressure is something that defies description. I also became aware of the evident failure of the mainstream medications which I had been prescribed. Since blood pressure is not a physical item, having the characteristics of neither an organ, nor a biological system, the medical community lacks the understanding to fully comprehend the beauty of continuous blood flow.

I do not intend to reveal or understand the reasons for following an imaginary tale to treat the health of the human being. I find that there are many important points to be made like the multiple billions of dollars industry dedicated to the production and sale of fake high blood pressure lowering medication to treat a fake syndrome. In fact the volume of high blood pressure lowering medication prescribed is one of the highest contributors to the excessive cost of health care in the US. The reason is that established danger level is actually the normal average pressure created by the heart as it performs its duty in fulfilling the requirements of essential body functions. I also have a personal stake in this discussion since my cardiologist tries to convince me to take blood pressure lowering medication due to my age and not due to my blood pressure readings, which he predicted would be going up. The catalyst for this book originated from a personal experience.

On November 2, 2014, while watching a live TV broadcast of Nik Wallenda's high wire walk across the Chicago River, I experienced the effects that stress has on blood pressure. In the period of two hours and 30 minutes, my systolic pressure rose from 140 mm Hg to nearly 200, as Nik Wallenda, was about in the center of the high wire 600 feet above the Chicago River. My pressure dropped down to 135 mm Hg in the next two hours. The diastolic pressure rose from 65 mm Hg to 110 and then descended to 80 mm Hg. The following plot is of the author's blood pressure readings produced by mental stress and anguish while watching a live performance of a dangerous act.

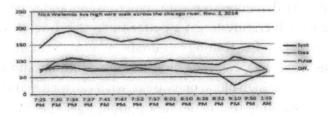

Author's blood pressure readings recorded during a live TV broadcast of Nik Wallenda's high wire walk across the Chicago River

This experience compelled me to gather information about the mechanics of the heart and blood pressure. After five years of research, I found that there is no consensus in the knowledge of the human cardiovascular system. Every author expressed his/her own opinions on how to interpret the makeup of the human cardiovascular system and its operation. The intent of this book is to describe the correct knowledge about arterial blood pressure and the findings revealed during this research. My own heart has been the main subject used to complete my research and reveal what I believe to be the facts about human arterial blood pressure.

I was surprised to find evidence of serious errors in the explanation the medical profession uses as a base to make their recommendations and guidelines, particularly when it bases patient care on the wrong opinion, an opinion which it has determined to be the correct one, but which turns out to be nothing more than a fairy tale.

This opinion is based on the belief in the existence of a false systolic pressure. The systolic blood pressure does not exist but the medical community is convinced that it does exists and that it carries a lot of information on the heart's condition. This can be easily verified by anyone with a stethoscope or just feeling and counting his own pulse. You start by counting the number of pulses your heart makes in a minute. The number you get will be somewhere around 60 pulses in one minute. When you check on your blood pressure you get two values per pulse - one called the systolic and one called the diastolic. Since the diastolic blood pressure is the pressure of the flowing blood, which is the other apparent pressure? This apparent pressure is called systolic and is the preferred pressure to be used for establishing the standard pressure guidelines for humans, even though it does not have an actual physical link to the human body.

INTRODUCTION

One of the many fairytales believed by the medical profession is the need for energy to inhale and exhale the air that we breathe. Conventional thought appears to be that we need a supply of energy to inhale the air and fill our lungs, but we do not need any energy when we exhale - supposedly because the air goes back to the atmosphere. The fact is that we do use exactly the same amount of energy when we inhale as when we exhale. The difference lies in the fact that the energy needed to exhale the air is stored in the diaphragm during inhalation and is used in expelling the air out of the lungs when exhaling.

Another fairytale is that hypertension happens when the maximum pressure value recommended for blood pressure, 120/80, is exceeded; yet this value is so low, it is actually in the approximate center of the normal operating range. Indeed, I found that this maximum pressure is routinely exceeded by most people during a normal working day without any visible effects. The medical profession currently uses health recommendations and guidelines based on a patient's systolic blood pressure. Nikilai Karttkoff discovered this along with the complementary diastolic blood pressure in 1905. (History of Spygmomonometer).

While there is a vast volume of information relating to this topic, there has been little attempt to systematically review the literature. Government and private agencies appear to have sanctioned the present beliefs without being fully aware that the danger of using the false knowledge and spreading it is by far greater than any expected benefits. The information available at the time was insufficient to make the correct scientific deduction. In fact, blood pressure knowledge has not progressed in the last 100 years and has relied on the same fairy tale that was used to implant it, without any investigation about its veracity.

The treatment for arterial blood pressure, as it is promoted by the medical profession, induces a patient to take blood pressure lowering medication until they are below a certain systolic number. The intention may not have been to create a fairytale. Blood pressure is not a physical item that can be set at any nominal value established by the American Health Association (AMA), World Health Organization (WHO), American College of Cardiology (ACC), or any other organization. The problem is that the medical community cannot imagine an item that is beyond description.

The following quote represents the most general belief as expressed in the 2017 updated guidelines by the American Health Association (AMA), World Health Organization (WHO) or any other organization:

> *Blood pressure is the pressure of circulating blood against the walls of the arteries.*
> *The Systolic blood pressure is the maximum pressure exerted by the left ventricle as it contracts.*
> *As the left ventricle relaxes, the arterial pressure falls.*
> *When the aortic valve closes, blood flow stops.*
> *The diastolic blood pressure is the pressure exerted against the walls of the arteries when the left ventricle is at rest.*
> *Remember that the top number is the systolic pressure, and the bottom number is the diastolic or resting pressure.*

While I did not know much about blood pressure, in my engineer's mind, it seemed to be highly abnormal that the ventricles were described as operating independently when they were mounted and operated by the same heart muscle that provides the energy to operate them. I re-read the same paragraph unable to understand how the ventricles could operate independently without any muscular source of energy. Then to my amazement, I read that the blood flow **stops!** Unable to understand, I was intrigued to research the blood flow system in search of the truth about blood pressure.

I learned that the blood flow cannot stop for an instant without serious consequences. What I found is that the whole paragraph was totally wrong. It does not represent the actual operation of the cardiovascular system. It appears to have been written by someone totally unfamiliar with control circuits in general and the human circulatory blood flow control system in particular. In fact all six sentences, are not true. Here's why:

The first sentence: *Blood pressure is the pressure of circulating blood against the walls of the arteries.*

Here we have two dynamic blood pressures to consider, the systolic blood pressure is a short peak at the start of the cycle that is not relevant to the flow, and the diastolic which is a dynamic pressure reading generated by the blood flow; it pumps the 6 L of blood to flow in the arteries of the main cardio loop. Both pressures may change with every heart beat and change according to the flow changes demanded by the organism. It is not a physical item with a mass that can be set at a value and expected to stay there. It is a pressure reading with a value generated in the time just prior to begin the pulse cycle. It is a static assumption that does not represent any of the heart's operations, it is not truly a relevant pressure.

The second sentence: *The Systolic blood pressure is the maximum pressure exerted by the left ventricle as it contracts.*

Systolic blood pressure is a peak produced by both ventricles every second at the beginning of the pulse cycle; It is a pressure peak that is not relevant to the blood flow volume or to any specific side of the heart; therefore it is not a true indicator of the hearts condition.

The third sentence: *As the left ventricle relaxes, the arterial pressure falls.*

This sentence describes something that does not happen; neither ventricle relaxes for the pressure to fall. The heart muscle is either compressing or expanding the ventricles once in every pulse cycle. There is no relaxing between the compression and expansion of the ventricles. During compression, the pressure increases by a few mm Hg above the diastolic pressure and decreases by the same amount at the end of the pulse keeping the blood flow constant in an unending flow.

The fourth sentence: *When the aortic valve closes, blood flow stops.*

The blood flow never stops in the human cardio system. The aortic valve is held open by the flowing blood, it closes along with the pulmonary valve when the flow is redirected by the heart muscle reversing from compression to expansion and returns to normal. The transition lasts about 10 to 30 milliseconds. The blood flow never stops. Neither ventricle gets a chance to rest, there is not enough time. The heart muscle does not stop, rest or relax; and was designed to be in continuous motion. That is why it demands a continuous supply of fresh oxygenated blood supply.

The fifth sentence: *The diastolic blood pressure is the pressure exerted against the walls of the arteries when the left ventricle is at rest.*

The diastolic blood pressure is the even pressure generated by the compression and expanding heart pulses prompting the resulting blood flow. Neither the left or right ventricle gets to rest. The ventricles are either compressing or expanding, but they do not rest at any time. The diastolic blood pressure is not affected and cannot be lowered safely by blood pressure lowering medication.

The sixth sentence: *Remember that the top number is the blood in a blood pressure reading is the systolic pressure, and the bottom number is the diastolic or resting pressure.*

The top number represents a meaningless pressure inconsistent with the heart muscle operation, and the bottom number represents the dynamic pressure generated by the blood flow as it fulfills the essential functions' requirements. Thus we have no choice but to discard the top number and refer the bottom number as the diastolic blood pressure generated by the beating heart which does not rest at all during its lifetime.

The diastolic pressure is the result of one well-orchestrated and precisely synchronized operation of the heart. The atria and the four valves that maintain the blood flow direction. The diastolic pressure is the constant arterial pressure present in the system due to the blood flow which is produced by the heart, which never stops. This diastolic blood pressure is directly proportional to the physical or mental activity the subject is engaged in. This is the pressure that occurs at the completion of every heart pulse, and reveals the present health needs of the organism. Diastolic pressure is the result of the blood flow in the cardiovascular system. This system distributes the nutrients and oxygen required to maintain life according to the needs of the organism throughout the body, as well as maintain a reasonably clean operating environment. This flow is controlled and adjusted by the blood-flow control system in response to the activities the organism is engaged in.

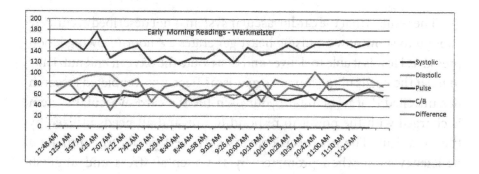

Early Morning BP Readings by Author

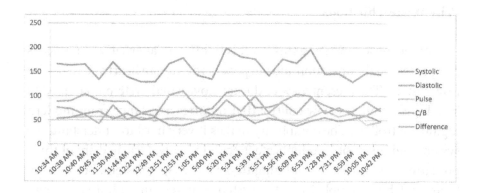

A Early Morning BP Readings of Author

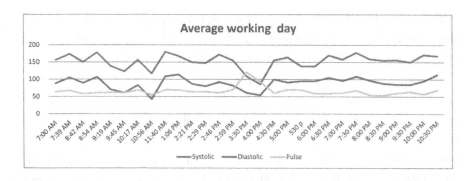

Average work day by author

The result is that the cardiovascular system is not described accurately enough to show how a pulsing heart generates a smooth flowing blood pressure. How is it able to deliver and distribute the oxygen and nutrients to meet the needs of the human organism? Recently completed research has unveiled that to maintain your own life the cardiovascular system is charged with the power to respond to any and all needs utilized by the organism. The organism delivers sufficient goods to eliminate a deficiency even when prompted by the mental stress and anguish experienced by an observer watching a live performance of a dangerous act on television from the comfort of their armchair.

Why Write This Book

My purpose in writing this book is to offer an alternative, engineer's perspective on the operation and purpose of the human heart and the blood flow system. The present view of the cardiovascular system is claimed to be a highly complex flow control that requires assistance from modern digital controllers. The complexity makes it very hard to understand the system and impossible to replicate it economically. I learned about three pressure control systems claiming to have the right system, but none of them match the simplicity of the system inherent in all human beings. Since none of the existing pressure control systems met with my approval for use in my own organism I had to find the correct control system in order for my cardiologist to come up with the proper care.

Aurora Health Care and many corporations involved with healthcare and body fitness have their own versions of how the heart is supposed to work. Aurora explains in detail, in their *Health Care Instructions,* the difference between *Left or Right Side Congestive Heart Failure.*

It starts with a short explanation of the physical heart components, describing how one main loop is split into two loops, each with its own ventricle, located in the right and left side of the main body. This is a misleading belief created by the assertion that there are two secondary loops, each one with its own pump. The fact is that the main loop is represented as two separate loops, each one independent of the other, even though they share the same blood flow volume. This shared blood flow volume together with the muscle power working both ventricles at the same time, is indicative of two single loops synchronized and working together as one single loop.

Aurora briefly describes the heart's purpose, which is to deliver blood high in oxygen content out of the right side of the heart and return it to the left side, from where it is pumped back out to the rest of the body. The cycle begins again with a return of blood to the right side. Aurora goes on to say that congestive heart failure happens when the heart is physically damaged not only on one side of the heart but eventually on both sides. This is very unlikely as each pump on either side is designed to carry the full loop load.

It starts with the right-side of the heart failure where a weakened heart cannot handle the blood it is getting from the rest of the body. Again, this is very unlikely as each ventricle is designed to carry the full loop load without strain. Blood collects in the veins and fluid leaks out into the tissues and gravity tends to collect this blood in the lower extremities.

The Aurora Health Care Instructions go on to claim that: *left side of the heart is weakened and can't handle the blood it gets from the lungs and fluid leaks in the lung tissues causing the patient to feel short of breath weak or dizzy.* This sentence leads the patient and medical professionals to believe that there are two independent pump operators. This is not true as both sides of the heart form part of one heart muscle; they operate together in perfect synchronism with a shared load.

The other error in that statement is the one claiming that the left side of the heart is weakened and can't handle the blood it gets from the lungs which causes the patient to feel short of breath and dizzy. That's another impossibility as either the left side or the right side of the heart is perfectly capable of handling the load coming from the lungs. In fact it is designed to handle twice the normal load of a single side.

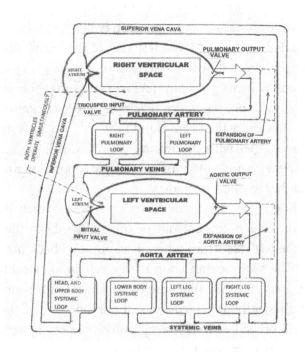

Both sides of the heart form part of one heart muscle; they operate together in perfect synchronism with a shared load.

The medical establishment of systolic pressure does not really represent any kind of a consistent method to serve as a standard pressure for ALL humans.

It is really the diastolic pressure that propels the blood from the heart to the body and from the body back to the heart. The diastolic pressure is the only source of energy produced by the heart muscle when it compresses and when it expands.

This pressure is utilized by the ventricles to get the blood moving. As it reaches the end of its travel the heart muscle switches to the expansion mode and fills both ventricles with the blood coming back from the systemic distribution loop.

The Importance of Blood Flow

Systolic blood pressure is the first pressure beat that can be heard when measuring the pressure with a cuff. It is a pressure that appears to represent a partial pressure generated by the physical flow activity. No one knows what it represents or what generates it. The systolic pressure varies between 80 to 200 mmHg in a normal day. This is the pressure assumed to be evident in the system. It is about 50 to 100% higher than the diastolic because it rides on top of it. This pressure is only an instantaneous peak at the beginning of the pumping cycle. Sometimes the systolic pressure appears to represent the compression force of the heart muscle. That is why it is known as the systolic blood pressure. However, these readings are so unreliable that the results cannot be trusted.

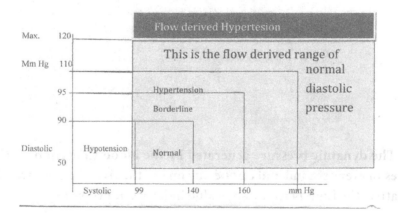

Flow derived Range of Normal Diostolic pressure

A PQRST wave results from an ecocardiogram (ECG). "The P wave represents the depolarization of the left and right atrium and also corresponds to atrial contraction. Strictly speaking, the atria contract a split second after the P wave begins. Because it is so small, atrial repolarization is usually not visible on an ECG." ECG." (www.aclsmedicaltraining. com.) has given the systolic pressure an unprecedented boost despite being based on an unreliable source. Also the ten or twelve lead computer tests appear to have become so popular due to its simplicity and the computer's ability to print out a detailed report on some ten or twelve different electrical signals from the left and right side of the organism. However the random placement of the electrodes on the front of the trunk area that is crisscrossed by many more unidentified signals than the ones selected, leaves their accuracy in doubt.

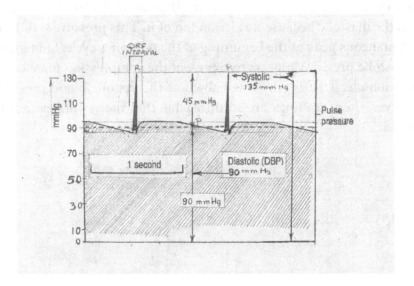

The dynamic pressure generated by the blood flow changes five times in every second and can be any one of the five, the positive, the negative, the high peak, or any value in between pressures.

Diastolic blood pressure is the second beat heard when taking the blood pressure of the arm. It is generated by the blood volume as it flows in the cardiac system and ranges from 50 to 130 mmHg which is the maximum that can be generated by the heart muscle under normal operating conditions. To perform this job the heart pumps the blood through a cardiac system at a flow rate that meets the requirements of the organism at the time. These requirements vary continuously according to the physical and mental activity the person is engaged in. They vary in humans from a minimum flow that generates a pressure of 50 mmHg to a maximum flow that generates a pressure of 130 mm

Hg. This pressure is called the diastolic. These pressures are produced by the blood flow volume and cannot be modified artificially.

The Case of the Blood's Flow (Hydraulic Flow)

The Cardio Circulatory Control system in the human body is the simplest, self-contained, economical and efficient pump control system ever known. Due to the plethora of operating conditions to which the living body is exposed, designed to operate successfully without failure under all conditions, the human control system uses positive displacement pumps which are powered by the heart muscle.

The circulatory blood system is an interactive organ system represented by two fluid loops powered by the heart, the pulmonary loop circulates the blood through the lungs where it is oxygenated by the respiratory system and the systemic loop circulating blood through the rest of the body to provide energy nutrients and oxygenated blood to every living cell in the body. These two fluid loops each represent one half of the main loop, but they share one liquid blood flow and one single source of energy.

The heart controls the blood flow by regulating the blood volume according to the needs of the organism to replenish it with the proper amount of oxygen, anaerobic and aerobic energy, including the nutrients to maintain its life. The potential aerobic (thermal) energy and the anaerobic (biological) energy provide the power for all instantaneous responses and sustained physical activities. They constitute the fuel that provides the power for the entire organism. The human circulatory blood flow control system contains a very sophisticated communication system around energy and nutrient distribution, including a sanitary waste collection and disposal system in one. It communicates with every single cell in the body and meets their needs to fill the requirements of the entire organism.

Understanding energy is critical to help understand my thoughts about blood flow. For this reason, I have divided this discussion into two books. Book One deals with the topic of understanding energy. Blood flow itself is discussed in Book Two.

ENERGY

What is Energy

While energy is a topic of another book all together, it is worth describing here since we are interested in knowing what kind of energy the human organism requires to sustain life and more specifically a healthy bio organism. Energy is the source of physical change in the universe.

Energy is the power that converts any physical mass, or an unanimated collection of physical masses that make up our universe, into a dynamic interactive cosmos. Living plants, animals and humans are the permanent evidence of the effect that energy has on inert mass. The science of thermodynamics is devoted to the study of thermal energy, the most evident form of energy. Although thermal energy, like all other energy forms, cannot be sensed directly, plants, animals and humans can feel the effect it produces when approaching a physical mass containing more or less thermal energy than their own.

One of the underlying causes of the problems with nutrition, health and diet may be related to the obsolete belief that we inhabit a purely physical universe in which everything just happens due to some inherent thermal energy, or other unknown causes. In fact Darwin's theory of evolution is based on the imaginary existence of self-powered physical masses which run around frantically in search of food and reproducing.

Scientists are well aware that the whole universe consists of something that is just as real as the inanimate physical mass which surrounds us.

We are all familiar with this "something" that has no physical presence but becomes evident by the physical effect it produces. The component I am referring to is so familiar to every human that it is taken for granted just like all the other physical mass that surrounds us. We tend to ignore its existence as a non-physical something and treat it only as another form of physical mass when we want to utilize it for our benefit. This component is commonly known as energy.

Energy is usually neglected, because it can only become evident by the effect its action produces on a physical mass. Energy is a non-physical power that affects a physical change, which appears in the universe, even though it cannot be perceived unless it acts on a physical mass.

Energy keeps the earth orbiting around the sun and maintains the earth's rotation on a non- existing axis. It exposes most of its surface to the life giving energy-rich rays of the sun, which is what prompts the growth of plants like grapes on a vine. Energy enables one to read the contents of this page and understand its contents based on the acquired skill of language (interpreting the sounds emitted to express our thoughts). There is no question that we are part of the physical mass portion of the universe. It is equally true that our physical human body is a dynamic system animated by the effect of a complex interaction of various energy types or functions. Without biological energy there would not be any living creatures on planet earth. Without anaerobic energy there could not be any rotating planets orbiting in the space between galaxies.

The abundant evidence of energy throughout the universe is undeniable proof that energy is just as real as physical matter. The issue with energy is that it does not possess any physical properties to become as evident as the physical universe on which it acts. Energy becomes evident only by the permanent or temporary physical effect of the change it produces on a physical mass. Physical changes are temporary, thus usually always reversible. The effects can be undone by reversing the energy unless it was broken or damaged. One exception is chemical energy changes which are permanent changes in the chemical composition.

Whether the scientific community agrees or disagrees with these statements does not change the fact that without energy the universe as we know it could not exist. Energy is not perceivable by the human senses because it belongs to the universe that has yet to be acknowledged by physical science; the **non-*physical*** domain I call Exmos.

Every physical change or modificatvion that can be observed in a physical mass is the well-defined effect of the action of some form of energy, or a combination of energy functions, acting on that mass. Without energy no physical change can take place.

The presence of energy can only be inferred by the observable effect produced from its application to the mass. This is an expansion on the principle of entropy in the second law of thermodynamics. This postulate in effect establishes energy as the cause of every observable change in the physical characteristics or features of a physical mass, invalidating the assumed concept of the occurrence of spontaneous changes as claimed by Darwin's Theory of Evolution. In effect the whole theory of evolution is based on the belief that a physical mass has the energy to grow and judge the correctness of the change it is going to make. All physical materials on this planet are inert; they do not have the energy to make a change in themselves, or in any other particle of physical mass, or to qualify the changes made to be correct.

The most common and obvious form of energy on earth exists from the beginning of time, and continues to exist in the commonly known form of gravity. The sun's combination of thermal and light energies is the next most common form of energy on earth. Next are the popular energy forms harnessed by man: chemical, mechanical, electrical, fossil fuels and nuclear energy, all following in close succession. The energy forms not yet harnessed by man are gravity, biological energy, time and life. Although these last three have not yet been officially acknowledged by physical science to be a form of energy belonging to the energy group, they are just as real as electricity because they are essential in explaining the existence of billions of living entities on planet earth.

Biological Energy

The physical universe in which we live is the product of the effect produced by the non-physical power called energy. The physical universe is the observable effect of the transformation of a potential power into a physical change produced on a mass. Energy in all its multiple forms is the natural originating cause of all the existing physical mass on earth, the planets, and the entire universe. Energy is what furnishes the power that we know as life in all living entities. Without energy there can be no animated mass on earth or the universe. Without biological energy there can be no plants, animals or humans. Energy is therefore the one component without which there can be no earth, no universe, not even empty space between the galaxies.

The entire universe is evidence of the presence of energy. The earth rotating around a non-existing axis in an elliptical orbit around the sun is evidence of an energy form that we still don't understand, even though we know that it has to be an anaerobic form of energy. There simply is no oxygen in space to generate any form of aerobic energy form. This forces us into having to accept anaerobic energy as being as real as aerobic energy. Yet the scientific community thus far has eluded acknowledging the existence of an anaerobic energy.

The universal presence of energy in all its functions has moved us into the false concept of assuming it to be a physical phenomenon. Yet every bit of mass is physically inert even though composed of atoms originated and held together by biological energy, or the energy form called the strong force. Any change in volume, position, shape, texture, temperature, size or consistency of a physical mass is the result of the action of some form of energy.

Energy is the Universal power that converts the static inanimate physical mass in our universe into a dynamic one, like the one we happen to live in. Living plants, animals and humans are the permanent evidence of the effect that biological energy has on inert physical mass. The science of thermodynamics is devoted to thermal energy, the most evident form of energy; although it is not the only one contributing to the dynamism of planet earth.

4

Without the addition or subtraction of some form of energy, any physical mass particle remains an inert particle forever. It is unable to change any of its physical properties like texture, temperature, size, volume, shape, color, position in space, and speed or direction of motion. For a physical change to become evident as effect in any of these physical properties requires the application of some form of energy.

The purpose of food becomes evident once energy is acknowledged as the foundation needed to sustain a living entity by replenishing the biological energy by consuming food. Without the ability to utilize biological energy to effect the physical change perceived as life, there could not be any living entities on earth. Biological energy is therefore the essential ingredient for any organism to grow, mature and multiply. Food is the renewable source of biological and thermal energy, which is needed to resupply the energy released from the food, utilized by animals and humans.

Thermal energy, even though it is presently believed to be the only energy that powers the living entities on planet earth, is not the only energy that sustains us. The anaerobic energy thus far not considered part of the human entity is called biological energy. This energy is utilized by every living creature to replenish the energy utilized in the living process. This process requires a constant supply of several biological energy functions to replace the ones transformed into a physical observable change.

The main energy source in use by all living species on earth— past, present and future —is the sun. Thermal energy, light energy and biological energy are emitted by this natural energy source. Once thermal energy and light energy acts on plants, it is stored in the living cells of growing plants for utilization by animals and humans in the form of carbon and biological energy. The combination of carbon, stored in every organic cell, with oxygen produces thermal energy. The biological energy can only be stored as an anaerobic energy source. Therefore it is available for instantaneous use.

Plant sourced food is the renewable source of energy that serves as the transfer medium from the sun by serving as the living receptors. Photosynthesis is a plant's inherent conversion system that converts the sun's energy into biological energy that resupplies the energies utilized by every living creature on earth. There is no question that foods can be perceived by our physical senses. Solid and liquid foods are ingested, digested, and discharged as liquids or a semi-solid waste. We are all well aware of the physical nature of the process. What we tend to ignore is that true organic food contains not only inherent carbon that can generate thermal energy when combined with oxygen, but also three functions of biological energy ready to ignite thermal energy to deliver the power required to arrive at the final product and maintain our life in the process. Artificial substitutes lack these functions and therefore are not considered food.

The energy form unique to living organisms which enables a physical living cell to become evident as a living entity is called biological energy. It is the prime anaerobic energy source for every self-sustaining living organism. Living entities are a physical mass of cells (one or more) with the inherent ability to show evidence of metabolizing food to extract the energy and nutrition required for growing and multiplying. Biological energy converts an inert physical mass into a self-powered entity that can move at will and feed itself to replace the energy it has consumed. It has to be resupplied with nutrients at regular intervals to sustain its health to grow and multiply into one or more copies of itself.

Just as the planets require anaerobic energy to go about their movements throughout the universe, so too the human body requires this force to operate within the design parameters. Anaerobic energy is derived from the three components of what we know as basic biological energy; Vitageny, Biogeny and Autogeny. I propose a fourth component that I call Remagen.

Vitageny is the one essential life sustaining anaerobic energy form in charge of directing, supervising, sensing and synchronizing all the actions of Autogeny, Biogeny and thermal energy in what is called the life cycle. It is the vital life support energy required to maintain all the control systems in operation and in perfect synchronism with one another. The physical effects of originating, growing, preserving and replicating observed in an organism, are products of Vitageny. Without biological energy containing the life function of Vitageny, the universe would remain an inert conglomerate of diverse types of mass in different forms. Vitageny becomes manifest by the observable physical effect of biostart (the original initiation of the reproductive process), metabolizing nutrients, growth, and reproduction evidence on a physical organism.

Death of any living being is a result of Vitageny stopping its function of enabling and directing the synchronized operation of all the control energies in a living organism. It is transformed into Autogeny and Biogeny functions to initiate and assist the process of biological decomposition.

The many billions of living entities in the world are self-sustained biochemical systems, because they contain Vitageny. Any attempt to ignore Vitageny is equivalent to explaining the operation of an internal combustion engine as a self-sustaining chemical system ignoring the fossil fuel energy that furnishes the power required to make the engine move. It is common knowledge that without the precise physical design of the engine with air fuel mixture systems and the thermal energy containing fuel it could never start, run, or appear to be a self-sustaining system. Life is the physical evidence of non-physical biological energy acting on a physical organism. The self-sustaining action of a physical organism is the result of a non-physical biological energy form executing all the control functions required to sustain the continuing operation of the living organism.

Even though Einstein did not state it openly, his revelation that the universe is the combination of energy and mass displaced Darwin's Theory of Evolution. Darwin was aware that without energy, whose presence he did not acknowledge, all mass in the universe is totally inert. The entire universe containing planets and spaces, plants, animals and humans is the merged result of an inanimate physical world powered by various forms of an all-encompassing non-physical energy.

Autogeny is the automatic functional energy responsible for the operation of all the independent automatic control systems within an organism. It is the automatic instinctive response energy capable of generating numerous predefined actions. These action depend on a number of variables sensed by the peripheral senses, or triggering the operation of a group of organs required by an animal to survive. It furnishes the preprogrammed power to direct an animal to search for food, consume it, move about, escape from danger and initiate reproduction. Autogeny also controls instinctive actions in a predetermined sequence when triggered by the signals received from the sensor system peripherals like the eyes, ears, taste buds, nose, feeling or the antennas of an animal or insect. It enables an animal to move about in search for food, recognize it as food, and eat it, defend itself from predators, and remember some of the repetitive actions that proved successful or not so successful in previous encounters.

In animals and humans, Autogeny is the energy responsible for maintaining the normal automatic uninterrupted and continuous operation of the functions provided by all the vital internal organs and control systems like the kidneys, jaw, tongue, heart, eyes, liver, cardiovascular system, respiratory system, immune system, nervous system, digestive system, growth control system, waste evacuation system, sensor system and the skin and body temperature control system. It has been loosely identified as the autonomic nervous system.

Autogeny controls the involuntary functions below the level of consciousness like sexual arousal, digestion, breathing, visceral functions, etc. It has also been identified as part of the sympathetic nervous system.

Similar to the BIOS program in a computer, designed to accomplish a specific set of tasks in a predetermined way, Autogeny is intended to accomplish a specific set of tasks automatically and repeatedly as required to maintain the health of the organism. Autogeny is the prime energy function required by all living entities to biostart, germinate, subsist, and move about. This energy cannot be generated by artificial means; it can only be produced by the action of the sun on the chlorophyll of a live vegetable plant. The plant extracts carbon and inert minerals from the ground, assimilates and converts the sun's energy into the thermal and biological energies for the delivery to other living entities in the form of plant-sourced food. These energies have to be continuously replenished in a plant to ensure the proper development and growth. It determines the direction of growth in a plant, down from the roots, and up for the stalks, changing course whenever an obstruction is met.

Autogeny has to be continuously replenished in an animal or a human to sustain the operation of all the control systems as long as it is alive. In animals and humans it serves as the power source for the independent operation of all the organs and control systems, such as the respiratory and cardiovascular system in order to combine carbon and oxygen for the production of thermal energy used to maintain a variety of specific duties assigned to the whole organism.

Biogeny is the cell's basic sustaining or maintenance energy that promotes the organized assembly of physical atoms into a single organic cell. It also forms the structure to bind many of them together into a multi-cellular organism. Biogeny holds and binds individual cells into an organized mass as one entity identified as a plant, an animal or a human. Biogeny is the power that enables a physical bit of mass to become a living cell by empowering it with the biochemical and organic substances required to have a predefined shape ready to be energized by biological and thermal energy. This energy is used to perform all the functions necessary to subsist, grow and divide under the direction of the information contained in what I call Remagen.

Vitageny is the life giving energy which acts as the organizing director of each physical cell which compose the living organism Growth and reproduction are accomplished by incorporating Biogeny which guides the growth and development of all the cells according to the construction specifications contained, in Remagen, for that particular cell. Remagen is defined as the genetic description and blueprint present in DNA.

Every cell in a group of cells shares the same genetic construction specifications as the other members of that particular group (bone, nail, teeth, skin, hair, muscle or a certain organ). Each group also shares some information about the construction specifications of the adjoining cells to maintain compatibility. Not every cell in the body has direct access to nutrition and energy carrying blood vessels. Every group of cells, therefore, has a nutritive substance and energy storage and sharing arrangement that enables them to benefit from the nutritional energy distributed throughout the body by the circulatory system (sap, or blood). Any damage suffered by a cell or a group of cells is reconstructed with the genetic information accessed by Vitageny from Remagen and implemented by Biogeny to rebuild the cells surrounding it. The continuous supply of Autogeny and Biogeny has to be replenished from a source that contains this form of energy. If a deficiency develops, the cell stops the growth process; it can no longer reproduce and dies. It becomes again an inanimate part of the physical world.

Biogeny can neither be produced artificially nor can it be replaced with artificial nutrient containing substances. Without Vitageny, Biogeny lacks the ability to make physical biological changes in a cell. Without any biological energy to grow, reproduce, and carry out all other biological program functions, there can be no life. The DNA information in Remagen, accessed by Vitageny, and the life sustaining functions of Biogeny, unique to a cell or group of cells, are essential for the support of a complex living organism.

Biogeny is the energy source that, when prompted by Vitageny, begins all the physical changes occurring in the cell of an organism. It enables cell growth and reproduction of all the cells and organs in a living entity as well as the maturation and reproduction of the complete organism. It becomes apparent in the ripening of fruits and vegetables. It is the energy that promotes the decomposition of any organic material soon after it is deprived of life energy. The short storage life span – freshness – of fruits and vegetables is due to the gradual depletion of Biogeny into rot or decomposition. It is also evident in vegetables which begin to wilt after they are cut off from the plant. It is also evident in the root regeneration when the severed plant is placed in water. The decomposition can be delayed by the removal of all the water content with the application of thermal energy. It can also be delayed by removing some thermal energy and dropping its temperature; this can also delay and even stop the action of Biogeny from continuing decomposition if dropped low enough. This is the reason that many fruits, vegetables and meats can be preserved for months by freezing at the proper time under the proper conditions.

The combination of Autogeny, Biogeny and Vitageny in the physical cells of a seed is what begins biostart, the germination process, to generate a new plant. The predetermined blueprint and specifications stored in the genetic code of Remagen are essential to maintain the exact reproduction of every single cell. Without acknowledging the action of Biogeny and Remagen there is no accurate scientific explanation of this process.

The presence of Biogeny does not alter the thermal energy content of the seed or substance on which it is acting. This is the energy that upon removal from the trunk of a living tree enables a hydrocarbon to dry out, retaining its entire thermal energy to become construction lumber that can last for an almost undefined period of time. This is the process that under extreme pressure and time converts the once living carbohydrates into the hydrocarbons that fuel our industrial revolution.

Aerobic Energy

Aerobic Energy requires oxygen to ignite and materialize, it is the result of combining oxygen and carbon. Unlike anaerobic energy, aerobic energy does this with oxygen to ignite thermal energy, or any other anaerobic energies.

Nine Essential Heart Functions

All cells, tissues, organs, and organ systems in humans are organized in nine levels according to the different heart functions that carry out the major body functions. The Cardiovascular Blood Flow Control System has the following nine distinct essential functions required to maintain the health of the various organs and the billions of cells in the human organism. The first two functions are well known and identified but the other seven are assumed to occur just when needed.

1. As previously noted, ***Vitageny, the Biological Life Energy Delivery Function*** is the most important function of all because without life there can be no brain, spinal cord and nerves that recognize and coordinate living cells, the muscular system, organs, or self-supporting organic entities. This function picks up biological energy from the digestive system and delivers it as the fuel demanded by all the cells, organs and muscles in the organism to be used to initiate the automatic repetitive, involuntary and/or voluntary organism functions (lungs, liver, kidneys, colon, urinary bladder, heart and reproductive organs)

in cells, muscles and organs that require it. The sensors in the blood are activated when they detect a need to refill the energy supply in any one of the organs or cells of the body.

2. *Oxygen Acquisition and Exchange Delivery Function* (aerobic) is performed by the pulmonary loop where the blood flow powered by Autogeny picks up oxygen from the lungs, exchanging the exhaled carbon dioxide collected from all living cells in the body, for fresh oxygen from the inhaled ambient air. The anatomical features of the respiratory system include the nose, airways, lungs, and the respiratory muscles.

   This oxygen-loaded blood is distributed by the second cardio-flow-loop throughout the whole systemic organism delivering life supporting oxygen to all the cells, organs and muscles; this oxygen is used by the recipient cells to combine with stored carbon to generate the thermal energy required for the execution of all the heavy physical and mental work demanded by a living organism. Autogeny, under the supervision of Vitageny, ignites the power of thermal energy to operate the muscles to expand and contract the diaphragm and the lungs at a rate of thirty to ninety times per minute to maintain the system's operation. All the living cells of this system are maintained by Biogeny. The lungs repeat the breathing cycle in direct proportion to the oxygen demand required by the various systems fed by the oxygen containing blood. This demand is due not only to the operation of the lungs, heart and other internal organs. It is also the result of any physical activity performed by the various muscles throughout the physical body.

3. **Circulatory and Digestive Function,** powered by Autogeny, picks up the same physical nutrients from the digestive system and delivers them as required to all the individual cells in the organism. It also provides the sanitary cleanup service functions to prevent unhealthy conditions. It picks up and collects all dead cells and other discarded waste and debris distributed throughout the living organism to be expelled along with the digested and undigested food waste from the digestive system.

4. **Growth Control Function** controls the growth of cells and organs, circulates the blood flow distribution system and maintains homeostasis. It is powered by Biogeny. It utilizes the structure of the hip, the pituitary gland, the thyroid gland as well as the pancreas to control the growth and development and metabolism of the human body. Whenever the organism is burdened by an excessive intake of animal sourced fats, protein and cholesterol, it overwhelms the growth control system forcing it to find suitable storage sites. Growth control will distribute equal amounts of cell growth to areas not confined within an assigned area. This will result in an enlarged circumference of the face, limbs, buttocks and stomach. Most internal organs as well as bones, fingers, and toes, are normally not affected directly by the excess fat, carbohydrates, protein and cholesterol; although they will increase in size to meet the needs generated by obesity or other repetitive physical activity. The uncontrolled growth of tumors and cancer cells becomes evident when a certain organ or tissue refuses to admit or recognize the growth control limitations from Remagen. Whatever causes this refusal is not yet understood by medical science. It is Biogeny, under the supervision of Vitageny, that will initiate the release of power from the thermal energy to maintain the systems operation. The blood flow control circuit regulates the blood volume circulated around the body. The blood picks up essential physical nutrients from the digestive system and delivers them as required to all the individual cells in the organism. It also provides the sanitary cleanup service functions to prevent unhealthy conditions; it picks up and collects all dead cells and other discarded waste and debris distributed throughout the living organism to be expelled along with the digested and undigested food waste from the digestive system.

5. **Disease Detection and Correction Function** circulates the immune system disease detection and replacement cells to maintain the overall health of the body and prevent the invasion of foreign bodies or infecting bacteria. Vitageny contained in the circulating blood picks up information about the physical

condition of every living cell and detects any damage or disease resulting from unusual conditions and informs the brain. The brain system controls the most basic functions of the body, such as breathing, blood flow, swallowing, and pupil constriction. Autogeny increases the blood flow to deliver immediate assistance as needed to correct problems whenever or whereever a deficiency is detected. The immune system also checks for any unusual conditions or physical impairments (cuts, bruises, or germs, thermal or UV radiation-produced problems). Autogeny powered white blood cells called T-cells are the hunter killers, scanning the intercellular environment for foreign invaders, locating and destroying cells of our infected system and eradicating cancer cells as well as activating other immune cells that manufacture antibodies. T-cells are in the forefront of our body's immune system defenses, present in both blood and tissue. They are unique to each person. The growth-limit control system utilizes the structure of the circulating blood, heart, blood vessels, hypothalamus, thyroid, and pancreas to control the growth of all organs in the organism. The growth and limit information comes from Remagen which contains all the standard dimensions for all organs in the proper proportions to match the whole. Whenever the organism is burdened by an excessive intake of animal sourced fats, protein and cholesterol it overwhelms the growth control system, forcing it to find suitable storage sites. The uncontrolled growth of tumors and cancer cells becomes evident when a certain organ or tissue refuses to admit or recognize the growth control limitation from Remagen, Whatever causes this refusal is not yet understood by medical science. It is Biogeny, under the supervision of Vitageny, that will initiate the release of power from thermal energy to maintain the system's operation.

6. **Skeletal Infrastructure Function** is the integumentary system (outer protective layer part of an animal or plant), e.g. skin, hair, nails, shell and bones system. It is the immune system disease detection and replacement cell system used to maintain the overall health of the body and prevent the invasion of foreign

bodies or infecting bacteria. The nervous system brain and spinal cord nerves recognize and coordinate the body's response to the environmental and circulatory system.

Vitageny contained in the circulating blood picks up information about the physical condition of every living cell, detecting any damage or disease resulting from unusual conditions and informs the brain. *The brain system controls the most basic automatic functions of the body such as breathing, digesting, blood flow, swallowing, and pupil constriction.* The immune system also verifies that there are unusual conditions or physical impairments (cuts, bruises or germ, thermal or UV radiation produced problems).

7. *The Intercellular Energy Access and Distribution Function* collects and distributes oxygen, energy and nutrients to areas and tissues that are accessible to the direct contact of blood flow from the cardiovascular system. The action of the Biogeny-powered intercellular energy and distribution system helps to regulate body temperature. This function controls the growth, operation, and metabolic development of every cell and organ in the organism.

8. *The Sexual Reproductive Function* is in charge of identifying the correct mate and arousing the proper emotions and physical activities to accomplish the reproduction of the species. This reproduction is external sexual and internal fertilization in the female. In the male it has two organs located on the outside of the body. The anaerobic energy delivery function can be initiated by the reproductive organs as they are prompted by the reproductive organ system and the imagination to be activated.

9. *The Excretory System is the Function* in charge of the process of eliminating metabolic waste from skin, lungs, liver and kidneys. The excretory system receives all the carbon dioxide from the respiratory system, eliminates the waste it receives from the digestive system and the cell waste from the circulatory system and in general takes care of discharging all the waste material from the body into the outside world. The skin, water, salts, and

a small amount of urea in sweat are continuously disposed of by the skin, even if we are not aware of it.

Every one of these functions is accurately performed by various organs and tissues in an organic system. Each function system has between a few hundred to several thousand sensors or sensing points distributed throughout the living cells of the organism. Whenever a sensor is activated or triggered into a flow increase request, it will utilize the anaerobic energy required to execute one extra pulse of blood flow required to fill the request. At the same time it sends a demand to increase the size of the right and left atriums of the heart to increase the blood volume delivered by the heart in the next pulse. This sequence may be repeated for several cycles until the increased blood flow has reached and fulfilled the demand for increased blood flow. When more than one function sensor is activated the individual percentages are added up to generate a blood flow increase that is proportional to the total required. The instantaneous response to increase flow is executed with the anaerobic energy in charge of operating the right and left atrium of the heart (the aerobic energy is not available for an instantaneous action). Both atria expand as they receive the signal to increase the blood volume to be delivered to the ventricles in the next pulse.

Of these nine essential functions, most or all rely on the replenishment of their energy by means of the nutrients in liquid blood, as delivered by the circulatory system. All function requests are cumulative, as they will add to any existing demand; they can add to an excessive large demand, resulting in a large flow increase request. The blood flow volume can increase by an increase in the pulse rate, the increase in the atrium of the heart volume, or by a combination of the two, a combination that can result in a normal diastolic blood pressure as high as 120, and a pulse of 90. Any diastolic pressure reading higher than **115** mmHg is a signal that there is some sort of blockage, hypertension or improper operation.

Every human depends on the correct operation of all nine functions to sustain the health of their organism. Any interference from prescription blood pressure lowering medication means a potential damage to the heart muscle and a reduction in the expected lifetime of the organism by the production fainting spells or dizziness that occurs from lowering the usual low blood flow volume for the relaxed organism. A low flow set point below the minimum required to sustain the needs of the organism results in dizziness, fainting and even death.

Due to the number of incorrect assumptions about the value of blood pressure in 95% of the cases of hypertension there is no evidence of a direct cause. This is called essential hypertension the direct cause of which, cannot be determined. Any attempt to lower it by chemical means will produce more damage than good. Attempting to maintain a pressure of 120/80 – 60 is a commendable pipe dream of just about all patients of low pressure medication - a value that can be easily accomplished sitting down and relaxing from whatever activity caused the elevated blood pressure.

For example, the transport of oxygen to the lungs and circulation throughout the organism is not the only job the heart is accomplishing. The heart is responsible for the proper operation of all nine essential functions utilized by the circulatory blood system to distribute the service throughout the organism.

Red and white blood cells powered by anaerobic energy act as health information transmitters, health care needs providers, waste collection and disposal, and emergency repair services for all the cells in the human body. Plasma is mainly water, but it also contains many important substances such as biological energy evident as sugars, glucose, protein, fat particles, nutrients, albumin, clotting factors, antibodies, enzymes, and hormones. All these substances are produced in the human bone marrow as part of the routine maintenance of the life containing physical body. Anaerobic energy ignites the thermal energy to perform all these cell maintenance operations. Iron containing hemoglobin is the oxygen-carrying protein that is found within all red blood cells.

Every human depends on the correct operation of all nine functions to sustain the health of his/her organism. Any interference from blood pressure lowering medication means a reduction in the low flow volume set point for the relaxed organism. A low flow set point below the minimum required to sustain the needs of the organism results in dizziness, fainting and even death.

BOOK TWO

BLOOD FLOW

The Human Circulatory Blood-Flow Volume System.

This is an interactive organ system consisting of two fluid loops powered by the heart. The *pulmonary-loop* circulates the blood through the lungs where it is oxygenated by the respiratory system; and the *systemic-loop* circulating blood throughout the rest of the body to provide energy, nutrients and <u>oxygenated</u> blood to every living cell in the body. The heart controls the blood flow volume through both loops by regulating the blood flow volume according to the needs of the organism to replenish it with the proper amount of oxygen, anaerobic and aerobic energy, including the nutrients to maintain its life. The potential aerobic (thermal) energy and the anaerobic (biological) energy provide the power for all instantaneous responses and sustained physical activities. They constitute the fuel needed to power the entire organism.

The circulatory blood system contains a very sophisticated communication system, energy and nutrient collection and distribution system, sanitary waste collection and disposal system, all in one. It communicates with every single cell in the body and meets their needs as required to fill the whole body's energy and nutrition needs. When exercising, the heart pumps harder and faster to provide more blood, with the lungs breathing faster and deeper to furnish more oxygen to combine with the carbon contained in every cell, igniting the thermal energy to operate the muscles. The increased blood flow also delivers more nutrients to support the individual hard working cells. During an infection, the blood delivers more immune cells to the site of infection, where they accumulate to ward off harmful invaders. All these operations are powered by Autogeny and thermal energy, controlled by and operated in synchronism with the signals from Vitageny, even though one is not consciously aware of any of these operations.

The white cells from the immune system circulate in the blood until they receive a hormone signal from the endocrine system that a certain cell or part of the body is damaged or threatened by disease. In response to these signals, the white blood cells leave the blood vessel at the damage location by squeezing through the blood vessel wall. They migrate to the source of the signal and begin the healing process by coagulating the blood to close the wound and form a scab or smother the bacteria to fight the infection.

Red and white blood cells prompted by Autogeny act as health information transmitters and simultaneously, health care needs providers, waste collection and disposal, and emergency repair services for all the cells in the human body. Plasma is mainly water, but it also contains many important substances such as biological energy, glucose, sugars, protein and fat particles, nutrients, (albumin, clotting factors, antibodies, enzymes, and hormones). All these substances are produced in the human bone marrow as part of the routine maintenance of the life containing physical body. Biogeny is the energy that ignites the thermal energy to perform all these cell maintenance operations. Hemoglobin is the oxygen-carrying protein that is found within all red blood cells.

The pumping action of the heart is controlled by Autogeny as it ignites thermal energy to operate the physical heart muscles. The heart of an adult is programmed to maintain the heart beating at a steady 60 pulses per minute at rest, speeding up during the day in direct proportion to the needs created by the physical or mental activity undertaken by the organism. The speeding up is intended to replace the energy and nutrition consumed by the small increase in physical activity or mental anxiety.

The cardiovascular control system is designed to let the blood flow gain access to every single living cell in the human body to deliver oxygen and collect carbon dioxide; it delivers energy and nutrients to all living cells and collects all the dead matter and trash; supervises the normal health of every cell and dispatches appropriate help whenever needed. It also communicates with all the other living cells and sounds the alarm if anything should go wrong.

To accomplish these functions the blood is maintained in continuous circulation within the piping system by the action of one heart which performs the two basic functions of maintaining a constant blood flow within the loops.

The two pulmonary loops from the first pump deliver the oxygen depleted blood to the lungs and deliver the oxygen rich blood to the input of the second pump; this pump delivers the oxygen-rich blood to the four remaining loops, and returns to the first pump. All these loops are connected in series, sharing the same flow and constituting a sealed, closed circuit with a constant supply of blood. The blood supply is fully loaded with hemoglobin containing red blood cells which have the ability to collect the oxygen and discharge the CO_2; they have aerobic energy and anaerobic energy to deliver any time it is needed. They carry the necessary hormones to heal any wounds or illness, as well as messengers to inform of the current status of the cells.

The Heart Muscle

The heart is a hollow organ about the size of a clenched fist; it is composed almost entirely of elastic muscular tissue and contains four cavities which are compressed and released every second by the muscle to maintain a constant blood flow throughout the life of the organism. This muscle, called the myocardium, generates a signal every second that initiates the compression of the ventricles before birth, and stops at the time of death of the physical body. The compression is the first of the two pump cycles which prompts the blood flow out of the ventricles and into the cardio piping system. In the second cycle the myocardium expands the ventricles back to fill with blood ready for the start of the next pump cycle.

This two cycle, compression, expansion, is repeated at least once every second or more, to maintain a smooth blood flow in the closed circuit piping system.

The myocardium is covered with a net of capillaries to ensure an abundant supply of blood. The contractions of the myocardium pump an average of 70 mL of blood through the circulatory system at an average rate of 60 contractions per minute. These contractions increase or decrease in frequency following the oxygen and energy demands required by one or more of the nine essential functions as a response in direct proportion to the mental stress and or the physical activity the organism is engaged in. These essential functions are described above in *Book One*.

The heart muscle contains two ventricular spaces, two atrium volume measuring spaces and four normally closed valves, which maintain a unidirectional flow of blood during the time that the ventricles are discharging their blood contents or filling back up.

The myocardium or heart muscle is more or less the same as any other muscle except that it is designed to operate continuously without missing a beat or allowing any rest 24 hours a day, seven days a week, and 365 days a year for 100 years. It also has the ability to force compression and release the pressure, (these are the only operations that the heart performs: compression and expansion). This permits the ventricular space to be filled again to get ready for the next pulse. It is designed with sufficient power to continue normal operations in the event of a failure of one of the ventricles, or a miss-operating valve.

Ventricular spaces are the two flexible cavities in the heart muscle that contain a normally closed input valve, and output valve. The input valves are fed from the atrium cavity above the ventricular space, the mitral valve from the left atrium, and the tricuspid valve from the right atrium. The output valves feed the output flow - the aortic output valve from the left ventricle into the four systemic loops, and the pulmonary output valve from the right ventricle into the two pulmonary loops trough the pulmonary artery.

Normally closed valves are in charge of maintaining the blood flow in a single direction during the muscle compression and expansion of the ventricular spaces. There are four normally closed valves to prevent the blood flow from reversing flow direction, but as long as there is one valve operating, the flow is unable to flow in the wrong direction.

Positive Displacement Pump

To understand heart failure it is important to know the sequence the heart muscle follows during the one second cycle repeated during the life of the organism. As the blood exits the ventricle space through the output valves it moves the blood in the direction of flow. When the blood is returning from the systemic loops and is filling up the ventricles, it also moves the blood in the direction of flow but through the intake valves. That is how the heart performs the duties of a positive displacement pump - by compressing the ventricles on the first half cycle, and expanding in the second half cycle.

This muscle has only one function to execute: to maintain the blood flow in the circulatory system. It squeezes the ventricle space to displace the contained blood in the compression cycle and expands as it returns to its starting position and fills up the ventricular space as it maximizes the movement of a new blood load. This operation is repeated every second during the organism's lifetime.

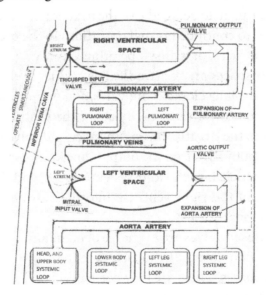

The heart muscle contains two ventricular spaces, two atrium volume measuring spaces and four normally closed valves, which maintain a unidirectional flow of blood during the time that the ventricles are discharging their blood contents or filling back up

Arterial blood pressure is indicated universally by a pair of numbers separated by a forward slash like 120/80 mmHg. The first number represents the high peak (systolic) and the second the lower maintained pressure (diastolic) of the heart's pumping cycle produced by the blood flow volume. The second dynamic diastolic pressure is the sustained pressure that distributes the oxygen loaded blood energy and nutrients to the entire cardiovascular system. A blood pressure reading is considered normal when the diastolic reading is within the normal diastolic pressure range between 46-120 mmHg, and with the heart beating at 60-100 beats per minute operating as a flow volume-adjusting pump that maintains a minimum flow of 6.1 Liters per minute.

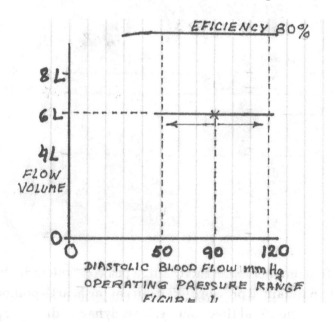

Normal diastolic pressure range between 46-120 mmHg, and with the heart beating at 60-100 beats per minute operating as a flow volume adjusting pump that maintains a minimum flow of 6.1 Liters per minute

Since the systolic pressure represents the peak of the pump cycle that lasts only a fraction of a second. The diastolic pressure is the one that represents the pressure that of the steady flow that distributes the energy and nutrients-rich blood that sustains the life energy in a human being.

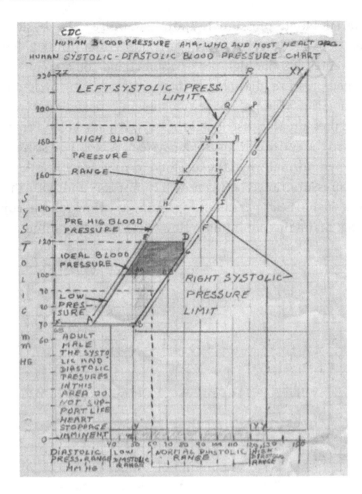

The first number represents the high peak (systolic) and the second the lower maintained pressure (diastolic) of the heart's pumping cycle produced by the blood flow volume. This dynamic diastolic pressure is the sustained pressure that distributes the oxygen loaded blood energy and nutrients to the entire cardiovascular system.

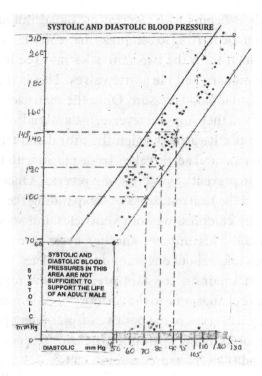

SYSTOLIC AND DIASTOLIC BLOOD PRESSURE

SYSTOLIC AND DIASTOLIC BLOOD PRESSURES IN THIS AREA ARE NOT SUFFICIENT TO SUPPORT THE LIFE OF AN ADULT MALE

DIASTOLIC   mm Hg

Human Systolic and Diostolic Pressure Chart.

Hypertension or high blood pressure is a term familiar to just about all people in the civilized world. We are all familiar with the stethoscope medical personnel utilize to listen to the patient's heart and breathing lungs to determine their performance. It is also used in combination with a pressure cuff to read the systolic and diastolic pressure produced by the beating heart. Although it does not really tell much about what the health of the patient being measured is, it is used by the medical profession as the first step in evaluating the health status of a patient.

Hypertension has become so familiar to everyone that no one is aware that it may be an erroneous concept. It is an erroneous concept for the simple reason that the systolic pressure is not a dynamic physical item with a physical body that can be adjusted and held constant at will. The heart adjusts the flow volume depending on the actual needs required by the living organism. It delivers the required blood volume with each heartbeat.

Each heartbeat begins with the timing signal initiating the cycle with the heart muscle starting to compress the ventricles which squeezes the loop with blood from the two ventricles into the main flow loop through the pulmonary and the aortic valves. This is the activity that generates the diastolic blood pressure. Once the ventricles have delivered all the blood content they stop and reverse, instantly admitting the blood flow from the respective atria through the mitral and tricuspid valves. The open pulmonary and aortic valves trade places with the mitral and tricuspid valves to prevent a flow direction reversal. Once the ventricles have been refilled the heart muscle stops expanding the ventricles and reverses, instantly compressing both ventricles and squeezing out all the blood content. This initiates another cycle of compression and expansion which takes about one second to complete.

The heart maintains a constant pressure flow regardless of the resulting pressure changes due to the various conditions encountered in the human body. This type of the positive displacement pump is clearly the only choice for its higher operating efficiency under a large number of operating conditions, pressures and viscosity.

The heart regulates the blood flow volume to meet all the functions that the organism needs to maintain its health. This is accomplished by controlling the blood flow volume delivered by the heart according to the needs of the organism: to supply, or replenish it with the proper amount of oxygen, anaerobic and aerobic energy, nutrients, immune system, communication, and sanitary services to maintain its life and health. The changing flow volume results in a large number of systolic, diastolic pressure and pulse combinations.

The diastolic blood pressure rises and drops in direct proportion to the physical or mental stress or activity the organism is subjected to. Therefore it may not be used or relied on to indicate any heart condition at all. The circulatory flow control system is in charge of fulfilling the requests of any or all nine essential flow functions. Any medication requiring the reduction of the blood flow demand will affect the organism's welfare.

The theory of the blood pressure control system was developed around the principle of fixed pressure operating characteristics. Today the evidence reveals that the present physical pressure pump is unable to operate efficiently at the various flow conditions demanded by the various activities that the human organism is capable of.

The difficulty of measuring actual blood flow forces the medical profession to measure blood pressure and accept it as a final evidence of a heart's efforts to maintain the life of the physical organism. The problem is that unless blood pressure is understood to be only an indirect intermediate result of the flow generated by the heart, it can be confused with a variable that has to be maintained at a certain fixed set point value. This is the exact opposite of what the human organism needs to remain alive and respond to the instantaneous needs created by variable present conditions.

The proclamation of any number of blood pressure combinations as normal, borderline high or hypertensive is an admission of believing in the fairy tale that the heart generates blood pressure rather than blood flow. It is for this reason that pressure is believed to determine the health status of the patient. The blood flow control system functions continuously without stopping during the life of the organism.

The purpose of the cardiovascular blood flow control system is to establish, control and regulate the blood flow volume needed by the organism to meet every one of the nine Essential Functions required by the organism to operate successfully. Measured by a cuff, The systolic blood pressure is usually about 50% to 100% higher than the diastolic because it rides on top of the diastolic appearing as a pressure peak - 120% to 160% or more of the diastolic. This pressure is the instantaneous peak pressure reached by the blood as it is forced out of the ventricles back into the closed circuit piping system. The use of the systolic pressure became common in the second half of the last century for no particular good reason. It does not carry any information and it can add anywhere between 50% to more than 84% of the diastolic pressure. Therefore it is useless in setting any standard minimum or maximum pressure.

At rest, blood flow is reduced to the bare minimum required to support life of all the cells in the organism. Due to the large number of variables involved, there is no one fixed pressure valid for all organisms. But a diastolic pressure below 48 mm HG in an adult male does not support life for very long, and death is imminent. Women and children have lower pressures.

Whenever the organism executes an instantaneous physical action requiring energy, it is performed by the instantly available anaerobic biological energy. When the heart is made aware of the need to replace the biological energy, it speeds up the pulse rate to increase the main overall blood flow to meet the demands and replace the used up energy. If the action is sustained for a period of time, the heart increases the blood flow to furnish the oxygen required for the aerobic energy to take over the action. The diastolic pressure is generated by the blood flow as the veins and arteries expand or contract at the end of the pulse. It also ignites stored potential thermal energy sending a signal to the lungs to increase the respiration rate required to meet the demand of additional oxygen.

Any reduction in the blood flow demand will reduce the pulse rate, reducing the flow between beats, followed by a peak overall pressure reduction. The cardiovascular system can be compared to a very complex service organization responsible for maintaining the continuous operation of all the organs, cells, and appendages of an organism required to maintain it in a healthy living condition. Since all the organs, cells, and appendages work according to their own needs, it does not make sense to limit the number of services offered by a static or artificaly reduced blood flow. These needs cannot be standardized according to a fixed schedule or operating load. The synchronizing action to operate all the organs at the right time and shut them down when done is executed by Vitageny, the life giving function of anaerobic energy.

When the body is at rest in homeostasis with the heart and the lungs at minimum demand and all other energy uses satisfied, the blood flow is as low as needed to maintain life in the organism. Any physical action requiring instantaneous energy expenditure uses anaerobic energy requiring an increased blood flow to replace the energy used in the action or activity.

The Pulmonary Loops

There are two pulmonary blood loops, one for each lung. Each loop receives half of the blood volume delivered by the heart. The pulmonary artery divides it into ever smaller arteries until the blood vessels become microscopic in size. These are called capillaries and in the lungs they are surrounded by tiny air sacs called alveoli.

The pulmonary loop begins on the output of the right ventricle and splits into two pulmonary arteries, each going to one of the lungs. After circulating through the lung capillaries where it exchanges the carbon dioxide with oxygen, the blood returns to left atria where it is adjusted to the proper volume required to meet the life function required at this time. This pre-measured blood volume enters the ventricle through the mitral valve and is forced out to the systemic distribution system through the aortic valve into the aorta. The systemic blood distribution system is made up of four independent flow loops that share the output flow of the aorta.

Where the alveoli and the capillaries meet, red cells in the blood give up carbon dioxide and pick up oxygen. Capillaries leaving the alveoli join into four pulmonary veins which deliver oxygen rich blood into the left atrium of the heart. This determines the blood volume to be pumped by the left ventricle in the next cycle.

After entering the left ventricular space through the mitral valve, this valve will close and the blood is pumped through the aortic valve into the aorta, the largest artery in the body. The aorta divides into four loops. This hemoglobin and oxygen-rich blood is circulated by the systemic distribution loops with many capillaries to distribute the oxygen-rich blood to every cell of the body. It takes about 60 seconds for a red blood cell to make the journey from the heart to the body and back again. During normal breathing operation the incoming air releases oxygen to the iron content of the hemoglobin and exchanges it for the CO_2-laden air from the body. This is an instantaneous operation.

The oxygen laden blood exits the capillaries and is collected by the veins that return to the heart. The left atrium expands or contracts to admit more or less blood into the ventricle. A contracted atrium allows less volume to be admitted to the ventricles, thus less blood will be forced into the cardio system. Since this is a closed system an adjustment must be made in the other half of the cardio system. In other words, the atrium of the other half has to reduce the blood amount pumped to match the reduction of this pump.

Upper and Lower Body Loops

The head, arm, and upper trunk loop receives about one quarter of the oxygen-rich blood discharged from the heart; the remaining blood volume is split in three equal portions to supply the lower body, abdominal organs, and each of the leg loops. The main arteries and aortas leading away from the heart have walls with strong elastic fibers capable of expanding and absorbing the pulsations generated by the heart. At each pulsation the artery and the aorta expand and absorb the momentary increase in blood volume. After discharging the blood volume, the artery and aorta walls spring back, maintaining the blood flow throughout the body until the next pulse. In this way the arteries act as dampers on the pulsating flow and thus provide a steady flow of blood through the blood vessels. Because of this, blood pressure varies continuously within the blood vessels during one complete beat of the heart - higher blood pressure with a peak during the first half of the cycle and a slightly lower blood pressure during the last half. These two unrelated blood pressures were known as the peak systolic pressure and the sustained diastolic pressure respectively. The diastolic pressure used to be related to the relaxation phase of the heart, but this is not really the case as the heart does not relax during its operation.

Due to this unstoppable blood flow, the lungs provide all the oxygen required by the cells to generate the thermal energy used to maintain the system in operation.

The carbon stored in the hydrocarbons, proteins and fat contained in every cell, is combined with the oxygen distributed by the flowing blood. It is ignited and available as thermal energy to take over the physical response to the activated sensors. When the increased flow volume reaches the area of the activated sensors with sufficient supplies to solve the problem, the activated sensor will shut down. The blood flow, however, will remain high, diminishing slowly until all the aerobic and anaerobic energies utilized in the action have been replaced and restored to normal; thereafter it returns to its minimum flow set point to maintain homeostasis. As a result of any request from another activated sensor, the heart responds by increasing the flow volume necessary to meet the new request.

The discovery that diastolic blood pressure goes up in response to the function demand, demolishes the numerous myths that exist about high blood pressure being the cause of cardiovascular problems and a large number of other health problems. Since the blood flow determines the steady diastolic blood pressure, this is the valid pressure to watch. The systolic pressure reading is only an instantaneous peak resulting from the expansion of the arteries and veins to receive the additional blood volume delivered by the heart; it has no significant meaning in the health status of the organism.

The removal of hypertension from the various assumed causes of the day will hopefully prompt health professionals to update their assumed reason for including blood pressure as a cause of almost all problems and will, instead, have them focus more on the actual unknown cause or original unknown source of the problem. The flow is controlled by a series of sensors distributed throughout the physical organism which activate the physical pumps to increase the flow volume in circulation propelled by the diastolic pressure.

Due to the large number of sensors distributed in the various organs, strategic locations, and extensive surface areas, it is normal for any human to have a dozen or more sensors activated at the same time. Under normal relaxed conditions, the average of various readings will result in a diastolic blood pressure average of **60-80** mm Hg as long as the body is not subject to a stressful situation. During a strenuous physical or mental stress situation, there can be many thousands of activated sensors. The average Diastolic blood pressure average can reach **110-90** under these conditions. This pressure, considered very high due to the 200 mm Hg systolic pressure reading, is completely normal when prompted by a combined stressful physical and mental activity, and can last for several hours after the end of the activity. When the energy, nutrient, and communication function consumption exceed the available supply, it can require two hours or longer before returning back to normal.

Every human depends on the correct operation of all nine functions to sustain the health of his/her organism. Any interference from blood pressure lowering medication means a reduction in the low flow volume set point for the relaxed organism. A low flow set point below the minimum required to sustain the needs of the organism results in dizziness, fainting and even death when sustained for periods longer than one or two minutes.

All the functions have to be executed whenever there is a demand due to some need. Otherwise the health and integrity of the organism is in jeopardy. Any attempt to interfere with the normal heart's response to a need, forces the heart to overpower the contradicting signals and work much harder in its attempt to meet the needs of the organism.

Pump operating cycle

The sequence of events is as follows:
Start of the pump cycle - the whole system fills with blood and the heart muscle generates the signal to start compressing.

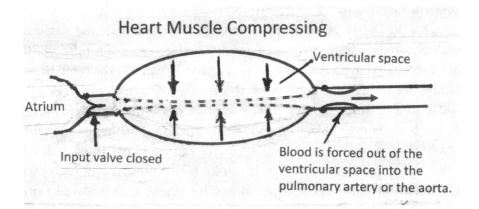

The heart muscle compresses the ventricular space and displaces the blood from the ventricles into the pulmonary loops and systemic distribution loops.

With the start signal the heart muscle begins compressing the ventricle spaces forcing the blood from the ventricular space out into the pulmonary and the systemic distribution loops. These loops are fed by the arteries and veins that connect them to the heart's ventricular spaces and are part of the closed loop. They have to increase their volumetric capacity by stretching their elastic walls. The displaced blood from the ventricular spaces forces the expansion of the elastic aortic and pulmonary arteries. This operation stores the energy as the diastolic pressure to be used during the next cycle.

The normally closed valves direct the flow in one direction only, by opening the discharge valves when it is compressing and transferring the flow to the intake valves when it is expanding the ventricles to fill them with blood.

During the compression phase, for the flow schematic of the complete circulatory loop. In the following section the same sequence is described as seen from inside the heart (as followed by the valves inside). The operation describes the inside of the heart as the normally closed pulmonary output valve is pushed open by the flowing blood being displaced from the ventricular space. This allows the blood to flow from the right ventricular space into the pulmonary loops and the left ventricular space into the systemic distribution loops. These loops, fed by the arteries and veins that connect them to the heart's ventricular spaces, are part of the closed loop and have to expand the volumetric capacity by stretching their elastic walls.

When the ventricular spaces are empty or have been discharged from all the blood, the heart muscle ends the compression mode by reversing back into the expansion mode, and the heart muscle switches into the expansion cycle to divert the flow from the output valves back to the input valves.

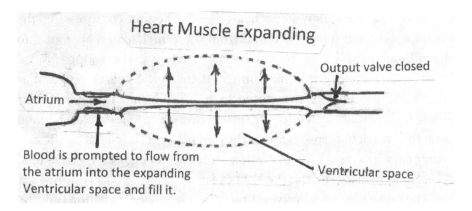

Heart Muscle Expanding

Output valve closed

Atrium

Blood is prompted to flow from
the atrium into the expanding
Ventricular space and fill it.

Ventricular space

The heart muscle expands the ventricular space prompting the blood from the pulmonary loops and the systemic distribution system to fill the ventricular space.

The heart muscle expands the ventricular space and fills it with the blood entering through input valves from the preceding atria. By opening up the ventricular spaces they receive all the blood flowing in through the input valves from the atria. The contracting pressure supplied by the previously expanded arteries and veins supports the diastolic pressure.

As soon as the ventricular spaces are filled up with blood, the heart muscle completes the expansion cycle by reverting back to the compression mode, ready for repeating the pump cycle. This operation is repeated every second during the organism's lifetime.

Inside view of the heart

The pump cycle is repeated continuously as shown in the typical example of five pump cycles in. A new pump cycle compression signal appears to be generated at the end of every expansion cycle.

The compression cycle starts when the heart muscle gets the signal to start compressing and exerts pressure on both ventricles to displace the blood they hold. The displaced blood pushes the two output valves (pulmonary output and aortic) open and initiates the blood flow into the lungs and the systemic system. This blood addition to the circulating blood builds up the pressure which expands the elastic arteries and veins to maintain the flow during the muscular expansion cycle.

The compression cycle ends when the heart muscle has emptied the ventricles from the blood they contained and reverses its compression to expansion mode. This permits the normally closed input valves to open under the pressure exerted from the elastic veins and arteries.

When the heart muscle stops compressing and reverses the output valves close and the input valves overlap. The input valves start to open as the output valves close When the output valves are fully closed, the expansion cycle begins. The heart muscle opens the ventricular spaces to fill them with blood. The ventricular spaces expand as they fill with blood rushing against the normally closed input valves which are forced open by the inflow of blood during the expansion cycle. As the ventricles expand they admit the blood flow from both the right and left atria. This flow volume is measured according to the needs of the organism and is allowed to flow into both ventricles filling them.

This cardiovascular flow control system is made up of a number of elastic veins and arteries that expand as the flow volume increases in the closed system developing a pressure peak; this causes a pressure increase slightly above the diastolic pressure which is accepted as the systolic pressure. Once the ventricle has completed its delivery, the veins and arteries contract and apply this slight over-pressure to the blood flow, maintaining a steady flow, until the next peak volume delivery.

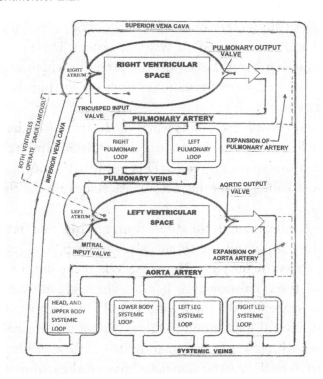

The contracting pressure supplied by the previously expanded arteries and veins supports the diastolic pressure. When the heart muscle stops compressing and reverses the output valves close and the input valves overlap, the input valves start to open as the output valves close, when the output valves are fully closed, begins the expansion cycle. The heart muscle opens the ventricular spaces to fill them with blood. The ventricular spaces expand as they fill with blood rushing against the normally closed input valves which are forced open by the inflow of blood during the expansion cycle. As the ventricles expand they admit the blood flow from both the right and left atria. This flow volume is measured according to the needs of the organism and is allowed to flow into both ventricles filling them. When the heart muscle reaches the fully expanded position it reverses ending the expansion cycle and starting a new compression cycle. This compression, expansion cycle takes about one second and is repeated at a rate of 60 times per minute. This cardiovascular flow control system is made up of a number of elastic veins and arteries that expand as the flow volume increases in the closed system developing a pressure peak; this causes a pressure increase slightly above the diastolic pressure which is accepted as the systolic pressure. Once the ventricle has completed its delivery, the veins and arteries contract and apply this slight over-pressure to the blood flow maintaining a steady flow, until the next peak volume delivery.

Liquid Blood Transport

Liquid blood is the transport medium utilized by the body to carry the oxygen, nutrients, communication and problem messages to all the cells in the organism. It also takes care of all the cleaning and collects all the waste that must be removed. It is used and reused over and over again. It is replaced with new blood when it fails to perform as expected.

Failure Mode Prevention

Ventricular operation, the utilization of two operating pumps.

In normal system design, I always include some insurance against the possibility of a certain failure disabling the whole system. To protect this cardiovascular system from total failure I would provide a spare pump to keep the blood circulating in case of main pump failure. But in the schematic diagram the original design already includes two pumps with two ventricular spaces. These two pumps are connected in a series on the one main loop, which means they both share the load of the whole system, and if one fails the other one will take over the whole system load. Since each pump includes an input and exhaust valve for the ventricle it already provides a spare valve in the event of the failure of one of them.

This means that the cardiovascular system for the human has been designed with a backup system in case the main pump or valve fail. I believe this protection against pump failure as sufficient life to the pump to make the whole system the longest lasting organ in the human body, even though I find that the medical profession attributes it to be the first organ to fail in almost 50% of the population.

CONCLUSION

Based on all the results of this research, I conclude that all the official printed material available through 2019 is deplorably deficient in presenting a believable view of the heart, the blood vessels and the human cardiovascular system in general. Due to the total misrepresentation of the physical components like the heart, arteries, their purpose and nonstop operation all the knowledge referring to be acquired over the cardiovascular system has to be updated with the knowledge revealed in this study.

The number of disclosures are so numerous and contradictory with the natural model as to be completely unfit to be used to modify the original pressure system, therefore useless for the purposes of establishing a scientific standard for blood pressure. The classification of hypertension into low medium or high, based on a systolic pressure number which appears to have little scientific rationale, not only has no application or use on a human system but confuses the real issue of health.

Blood Pressure Lowering Medication

The number of people whose life is affected by the misapplication of the blood pressure lowering medication based on the present pressure control system covers almost all the inhabitants of the earth. The reason is that the World Health Organization (WHO) and American Medical Association (AMA) dominate the world's knowledge of the cardio pressure control system. Around the year 2003 The European Society of hypertension (ESH), the European Society of cardiology (ESC) and the international Society of hypertension (ISH) decided not to produce their own guidelines on the diagnosis and treatment of hypertension but to endorse the guidelines on hypertension issued by WHO and AMA guidelines. These are the guidelines currently in place for most of the industrialized world.

The FDA claims to have valid clinical trials for the blood pressure lowering medications. They are invalid claims that should be verified. Politicians should initiate laws against the illegal sale of prescription blood pressure lowering medications instead of fighting marijuana which has at least some valid medical applications. Despite the ineffectiveness in lowering blood pressure, blood pressure medication is usually prescribed liberally as the first line of defense against many other diseases. They may have minor beneficial effects, but dangerous long term side effects that kill the patient in ten or twenty years depending on the dosage.

Due to the total misrepresentation of the physical, components like the heart, arteries, their purpose and nonstop operation all the knowledge referring acquired over the cardiovascular system has to be updated with the knowledge revealed in this study. Considering that the difference between the real flow control system and the imaginary pressure control followed by the medical establishment during the last 100 years is so large as to require a completely new project with a new description of a complete flow control system. The quality of care that any physician can deliver to his patients is based on the basic knowledge he acquired in medical school, therefore based on the application of the principles he learned. If he has an imaginary version of a pressure control system his patient care will not apply to a real physical patient with a flow control, but to an imaginary one. Some of the oxygen will be used to transform and deliver the thermal energy from the carbon into an aerobic energy to support the heart and lung muscles to replace the anaerobic energy. It also transfers all the aerobic energy from storage locations in the organism to replace the one utilized in the last run.

In the end, everyone must make the decision of what they believe and how best to manage their health. At the same time it is important to question long-standing practices that feel out of step with our own experience. The science of health, particularly of heart-health, has been studied for centuries and will continue well into the future.

APPENDIX

The following pages are devoted to a very small sample of the currently available printed material confirming our theory and opposing it. Although not customary in most books, I find it helpful to report in a clear and succinct way, what is true and what is fallacy.

The circulatory blood flow control system is in charge of fulfilling the requests of any or all nine Essential Flow functions. Any medication requiring the reduction of the blood flow demand will shorten the life of the heart.

The theory of the blood pressure control system was developed around the principle of fixed pressure pump operating characteristics. Today the evidence reveals that the physical pressure pump is unable to operate efficiently at the various flow conditions demanded by the various activities that the human organism is capable of. The pumping capacity of a positive displacement pump is essential for a human.

The real function of blood pressure on a human organism continues to remain a mystery. Medical professionals have been and continue to be trained on the conviction that a constant blood pressure is essential to maintain a constant blood flow. A concept that may be true under static unchanging conditions, the human organism, however, is designed to operate under a large number of undefined conditions that invalidate the original static unchanging conditions concept. These conditions include a range from restful sleep, to full-out physical and mental activity until exhaustion. All of these conditions can only be met by a positive displacement pump.

The Cardiovascular blood flow system is the only means in the human organism that can transport, deliver, collect, or inform about all its needs in any one instant.

Blood flow is the means utilized by the organism to distribute the oxygen from the lungs required by the living cells to survive, collect carbon dioxide from the cells and exchanging it with fresh oxygen. The oxygen demand is a dependent variable that has to meet to oxygen needs of the organism to make-up the increased consumption for all nine essential functions.

Blood flow is the means utilized by the organism to collect biological energy, thermal energy and nutrients from the digestive system distributing them to all the living cells and storage locations in the organism.

Blood flow is the means for the organism to perform the sanitary maintenance and disposal service throughout all the living cells and control systems.

Blood flow is the means utilized by the immune system to maintain the health of every cell in the organism by circulating the health information transmitters, collect and distribute corrective measures.

- Blood flow is one of many communication systems in the organism. Increasing the flow in direct response to any energy demanding effort, and delivering supplies wherever needed. Each one of these blood flows generates a large number of blood pressures. Each of the pressures is the result of the pressure generated by the blood volume as it flows through the blood vessels in the particular location of the test.

- It is physically impossible for a simple centrifugal pump to maintain all the health parameters required by the organism to survive successfully, without a complex blood flow volume control system. Every one of the following activities requires a higher blood flow which can be manifested and observed as an apparent pressure increase:

- The lungs have to deliver more oxygen to the blood to make up for any increase needed by the body due to physical activity or exercise. The blood has to travel through the body to reach the muscles being exercised and deliver the added volume of oxygen needed.

- Blood has to supply more energy and nutrients to the organism to replace the energy consumed during normal physical or mental activities.
- The blood has to fight infections by increasing the number of immune fighters to deter the spread of infections.
- The blood flow has to increase the delivery of white blood cells to help coagulate the blood and stop the loss of blood due to an open wound.
- The blood flow is one of the main or principal communication mediums between the brain and all the individual cells in the body. It delivers the complete status report on its condition.
- Blood flow is the vehicle employed by the immune system to deliver the clotting and bacterial infection fighting substances to whatever body area that needs it.
- The blood flow is in charge of collecting and eliminating all dead cells and other debris to maintain sanitary conditions, which increases with physical activity.
- A mental stress requires a large dose of oxygen for the brain to function properly.
- A sudden threat to life. Also requires immediate increase in oxygen supply preparing for the fight or flight.

Some of the incorrect conclusions due to the obsolete and incorrect assumptions and beliefs:

1. "A bigger waist increases your risk of developing metabolic syndrome (a cluster of factors, including high *blood pressure* and cholesterol, which in turn raises the chances of heart disease and stroke."
2. "Manage *blood pressure* (lower than 120/80 mm Hg) is one of the simplest seven lifestyle factors to take in order to reduce the risk of heart disease."
3. "Three quarters of the salt in your diet comes from processed foods, so sub in fresh whole foods to lower your *blood pressure*".
4. Scientists cited "increases in stroke risk factors including *hypertension* in younger patients".

5. "Regular meditation can improve your range of mental health measures as well as benefiting heart health by lowering the *blood pressure* and cholesterol levels."

6. "Monitoring salt and sugar intake if you have high *blood pressure* or heart failure . . . . . But sugar from high carbohydrate foods, also contribute to obesity, large waists, diabetes. . . . ., And *blood pressure*, all of which leads to heart disease.

7. Heart failure also can result from disease, high *blood pressure,* a heart defect present from birth, or symptoms of the heart muscle called cardiomyopathy.

8. "USDA researchers reported a study in which cranberry juice or a placebo beverage was given to 56 healthy adults. After eight weeks the cranberry juice group showed an average drop of 3 mm Hg in *both systolic and diastolic blood pressure,* while those on the placebo saw no change." *Fact: This is a typical farce common to all clinical studies on blood pressure. The 3 mm Hg drop in the systolic and diastolic blood pressures in a period of eight weeks. In eight weeks the patient's blood pressure has risen and fallen more than 3 mm Hg at least one thousand times unless the patient was in a coma and did not engage in any physical or mental effort. Apparently the testing personnel failed to observe this.*

9. "Longer commutes than 20 miles per day are associated with higher blood pressure, more worrying, and chronic stress, a study in commuting and health shows."

10. Normal pulse ranges from "50 to 76 b/m at rest. A gain of just 10 b/m over normal increases your risk of dying from heart disease by 10 to 18%," a study finds. *Fact:* The lower limits of pulse and diastolic pressure are not mentioned as if they had no importance at all, ignoring the fact that blood pressure lowering medication can drive down a patient's pulse to less than 50 b/m and diastolic pressure below the limit of 48 mm Hg. If it does the patient's heart will stop and he'll be well on his way out of the physical world.

11. "Most cases of kidney damage in the US are related to *high blood pressure* and diabetes. *Excessive blood pressure* damages

the delicate filtering member mechanism, and high blood sugar levels cause the kidneys to filter more blood than normal."[**Fact:** *Since high blood pressure is based on a fictitious number well within the normal operating range of blood flows, this statement is false.*

12. "In the general population aged 60 years or older, initiate pharmacologic treatment to lower blood pressure at systolic blood pressure (SBP) of 150 mm Hg or higher or diastolic blood pressure of (DBP) 90 mm Hg or higher and treat to a goal SBP lower than 150 mm Hg and goal DBP lower than 90 mm Hg. **Fact:** A *totally unfounded statement based on fictitious numbers.*

13. The difference between a blood pressure obtained from a blood pressure cuff on the arm and, an Ankle Brachial Index (ABI) from an ultrasound device on the ankle may require a stepped-up exercise program or a change in diet/medication. **Fact:** *Since it is perfectly normal for blood pressure to register different pressures in different locations this is a false statement.*

14. Drinking cocoa increases blood flow to the brain, because cocoa has sky-high concentrations of anti-oxidants called flavonoids which possess strong brain protecting properties. **Fact:** *An assumption that is impossible to prove.*

15. High blood pressure is blamed to be a possible cause of tinnitus, a sensation of noise in one or both ears. **Fact:** *Since high blood pressure is based on a fairy tale it can be believed only by fairy tale characters.*

16. High blood pressure is a serious medical issue, as it can cause heart and kidney disease and is closely linked to some forms of dementia. **Fact:** *Since high blood pressure is determined by fictitious numbers, this statement is totally without a scientific base.*

17. If not controlled high blood pressure can lead to increased risk of stroke, heart attack, heart failure, kidney failure and blindness. **Fact:** *Since high blood pressure is determined by a fictitious number. This statement is totally false without a scientific base.*

18. Globally, around 22% of adults aged 18 and over, have had raised high blood pressure in 2014. The mean systolic blood pressure of

the world population has stayed constant at 124 mmHg between 2010 and 2014. **Fact:** *Since the numbers for high blood pressure are based on wrong assumptions and determined by fictitious numbers, this statement is totally false and without a scientific base.*

According to the list of diseases, ailments or health problems listed above it appears that just about every treatment when heart failure risk is diagnosed solely on the present interpretation of systolic and diastolic blood pressure readings, it may not need to be treated as a serious medical issue. For high blood pressure is an imaginary condition based on systolic and diastolic pressure numbers that are surpassed every day while performing normal physical and or mental activity.

Normal blood pressure readings change continuously throughout the day ranging from low to high; therefore, they can be timed to prove conclusively anything that needs to be proven. It is for this reason that some patients continue to decline despite appropriate (by current standards) medical and/or surgical therapy.

Since there is no easy way to confirm the veracity of these claims, they are considered to be true. The problem is that the flow of blood to the brain is an independent variable controlled by the nine functions required by a living organism, rather than respond to transient physical changes. The notion that a constant blood pressure reading is essential to maintain a healthy heart and prevent it from causing numerous health problems is pervasive throughout the American medical profession. Just as it is throughout the world's health organization in all the rest of the world. There is however, some disagreement, "Hi, My name is Dr. Marlene Merritt (LAc, DOM(NM), ACN) and if you have high blood pressure, I BEG you... please don't subject your body to the toxic concoctions the pharmaceutical companies are trying to shove down your throat."

Another dissenting opinion comes from Dr. Sherry A. Rogers M.D. in her book "*The High Blood Pressure Hoax.* These two voices denouncing the High Pressure Hoax, do not know the real reason, or he whole story behind this hoax; they only know from their experience that what they have been taught is not true. Nearly all printed knowledge available today refers to blood pressure as if it was a goal to be maintained at or near the average value of 100 to 140 mmHg (systolic). A pulse of 60 beats per min is considered normal in adults with an accepted average of 72, rather than a variable that changes continuously in direct proportion to the blood flow generated to meet the physical and or mental activity of the physical organism.

- The continuous variability of blood pressure readings from one instant to another destroys the possibility of timing them according to a fixed time schedule or random isolated checks, or to consider them to be an accurate rendition of the Heart's physical condition.
- Blood pressure is believed to be generated by the pumping heart in response to the nervous sympathetic system that prepares the body for intense activity. This pressure is believed to prompt the heart to create the required changes required to meet the body's life sustaining functions. [Explained in the text] The trouble is that without an information link to all the cells that make up the organism, the sympathetic system is functionally unable to be aware of the organism's needs or the heart's performance at any one instant of time.
- Diastolic blood pressure is a measurement of the pressure generated by the continuous blood flow as it circulates in the cardiovascular system in response to one or more activated blood flow functions.
- Any instantaneous diastolic blood pressure reading reveals the heart's response to the blood flow needs of a requesting function, or a combination of various functions at that particular instant.
- To diagnose hypertension due to a normal occasional systolic high pressure reading does not make any sense. Prescribing any blood pressure lowering medication based on such a reading, will work against the heart's specific functions of increasing the blood flow to meet the organism's needs. In essence promoting heart damage and early failure. [Explained in the text]
- The cardiovascular blood flow system is a physical closed-circuit liquid conveyance system split into two main flow circuits. One

is the pulmonary flow from the heart to the lungs and back, and the second distributes the oxygenated flow from the heart to the entire organism and back again. Both of these flow circuits share the same blood flow volume as it circulates by the action of two separate positive displacement pumps mounted side by side in a single heart organ, synchronized to operate simultaneously as one heart, and supply all the life sustaining functions required as essential for a living organism to maintain its life.

- The entire human organism is powered by energy. There is no question about this, even though it is a known fact that there are two types of energy, each one with its own operating characteristics. The anaerobic energy that does not require any oxygen to act, is the only one capable of reacting instantaneously to a sudden need for power. Aerobic energy that generates thermal energy by combining oxygen with the carbon contained in all organic living organisms is the one responsible for the long term extended muscular operation.

- The flow is regulated by a simple Off-On Fuzzy logic control system responding to one or more demands for a flow increase to meet the ever changing oxygen and other functional needs required by a living organism. [explained in the text]

- Living cells take the energy from the ingested food through a series of bio-chemical processes called metabolism. During metabolism each cell combines carbon, nutrients and oxygen producing aerobic thermal energy, water and waste products. There is no anaerobic energy source identified. Even though it is the essential energy required to sustain life.

GLOSSARY

Aerobic Energy   requires oxygen to ignite and materialize. Unlike Anaerobic energy which does this without Oxygen to ignite anaerobic energy.

Anaerobic Energy   contained in the circulating blood picks up information about the physical condition of every living cell, detecting any damage or disease resulting from unusual conditions and informing the brain.

Atrium   One of the two blood volume measuring spaces built into the heart muscle. Atria is the plural of atrium.

Autogeny   The automatic functions energy responsible for the operation of all the independent automatic control systems within an organism.

Biogeny   Anaerobic energy in charge of controlling the growth, development and metabolism of the human body.

Cell   The basic structural unit of a function in living things. The power of living cell is provided by Autogeny.

Diastolic blood pressure	The second beat heard when measuring the blood pressure from the arm. It is generated by the blood flow as it flows in the cardio system and ranges from 50 to 130 mmHg which is the maximum that can be generated by the heart muscle.
Energy	The universal power that converts the static inanimate physical mass in our universe into a dynamic one, like the one we happen to live in. The Power required to actually perform the action required by the function.
Exmos Energy Theory	The science of energy. (Fred A. Werkmeister E.E. Kindle) 2015
Gas Exchange	The carbon dioxide produced by the cells that is transported by the circulating blood to the lungs. When we exhale we are secreting the carbon dioxide with a small amount of water vapor.
Heart Muscle	This muscle has one function to execute, it squeezes the ventricle space to displace the contained blood, and expand as it returns to its starting position and fills up with a new blood load.
Integumentary	The outer protective layer part of an animal or plant (e.g. skin, hair and nails, bones and oil glands system).
Muscle tissue	All body movements utilize biological energy to carry out a physical displacement or movement of the bones, organs or nutrients. Many are controlled by the human and the organism, but the majority react only to organisms request.
Organs	A collection of different tissues that work together for a specific function or sequential functions to accomplish their purpose.

Systolic blood pressure The first beat heard when measuring the blood pressure from the arm. It ranges from 60 to 210 mm Hg.

T-cells Are in the forefront of our body's immune defenses, present in both blood and tissue. They are unique to each person.

The kidneys A pair of fist-sized organs located on either side of the spinal column near the lower back. Through a complex filtering process the kidneys remove excess water, urea and metabolic waste from the blood. The kidneys produce and excrete the waste product known as urine.

The liver The organ that converts potentially dangerous waste products of protein breakdown into less toxic urea, the urea which is highly soluble is then transported through the blood to the kidneys for elimination from the organism.

Tissues A group of cells that perform a single function is called a tissue.

Ureters Transport urine from the kidneys to the urinary bladder, where it is stored until it is released through the urethra.

REFERENCES

"Advanced Heart Failure and Congestive Heart Failure" Medical Services : Academic-Community Medicine in South Eastern Wisconsin (Froedtert Hospital 2015).

Alice H Lichtenstein, DSC director of Tufts's HNRCA Cardiovascular Nutrition Laboratory

Biology: Miller and Levine (Kenneth R. Miller and Joseph S. Levine. Pearson Education Inc. 2010)

Cincinnati/Northern Kentucky stroke study

Duke Medicine Health News, August 2015.

Exmos Energy Theory: The science of energy. (Fred A. Werkmeister E.E. Kindle) 2015

"Healthy You" article (AARP magazine, February-March 2015)

Heart Failure :Advances in Prevention and Treatment. (Editors of Heart Failure in conjunction with Cleveland Clinic, 2014)

Jeffrey Blumberg, PhD, director of Tufts HNRCA Antioxidants Research Laboratory.

New recommendations for treatment of Hypertension. (National Institutes of Public Health-funded group of experts, JNC 8. 2014)

Outdoor Emergency Care (American Academy of Orthopaedic Surgeons, 2003) Jones and Bartlett Publishers. Sudbury, MA. 2003

Stanford University School of Medicine.

EPILOGUE

My father's final months and years, passed compiling data and presenting it in *The Truth About Blood Pressure*. For many reasons, I wish my father were here to write this epilogue himself. He would have known better how to structure his manuscript, layout his hand drawn figures and tell us what, in the end, caused his positive displacement pump to stop.

My father's heart stopped beating in hospice, August 23, 2019 at 3 AM, surrounded by those who love him. There was a nurse assigned to his case who administered medication to help him breath and dull his pain. His penultimate words to me were, "The book is finished!" I promised to have it published. His last words were, "If my heart stops, I guess I was wrong."

The first medication they gave my father to dull his pain, his body rejected, the reaction only made things worse. The second medication quickly sent him off to the sleep he was promised after peacefully having said goodbye to all his loved ones. My father's heart stopped beating in his sleep the next evening.

He died believing that his heart would not be the first organ to fail as long as his body was permitted to perform its basic bodily functions (such as blood pressure regulation) free from artificial intervention including over prescribed medication.

In the end the pain medications he received caused his kidneys to fail and ultimately his heart. One thing my father was right about---was perhaps not the organ itself, but his heart remained strong.

With heart full memory - Fred Jr.

Printed in the United States
By Bookmasters